With LOVE this book is dedicated to:

AURELIA

MADELYN

EMELIA

AUGUSTA

JULIA

Each of you are a beautiful ray of sunshine.

Big, COLORFUL raindrops are falling fast.
Surely this has never happened in the past.

Dropping like fresh fruit from the sky down.
Creating beautiful puddles to splash around town.

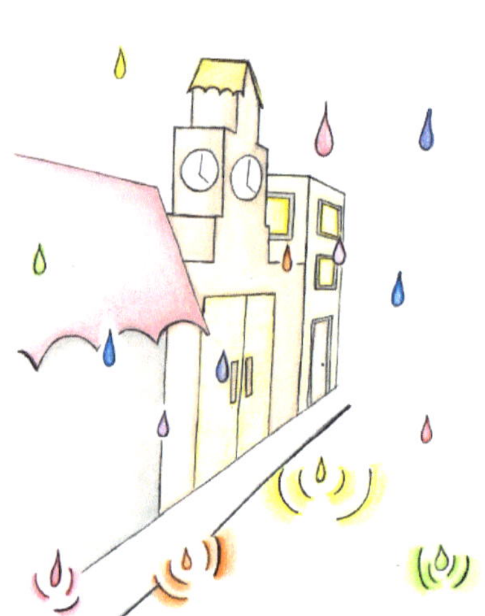

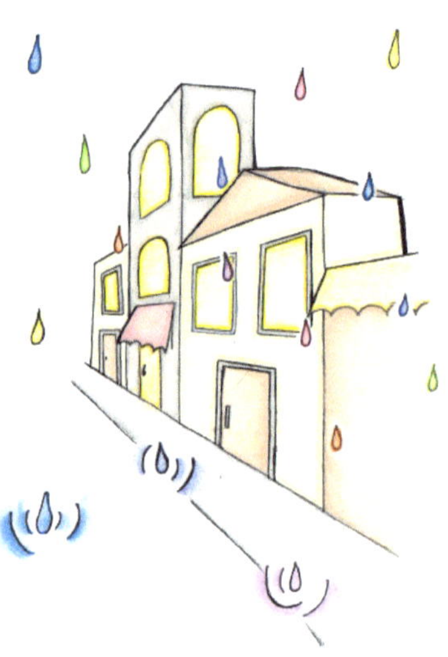

Drops of cherry red, banana yellow and berry blue,
fell with green, orange and plum purple too.

Something in the world is odd and funny.

Because it's raining and it's still very sunny.

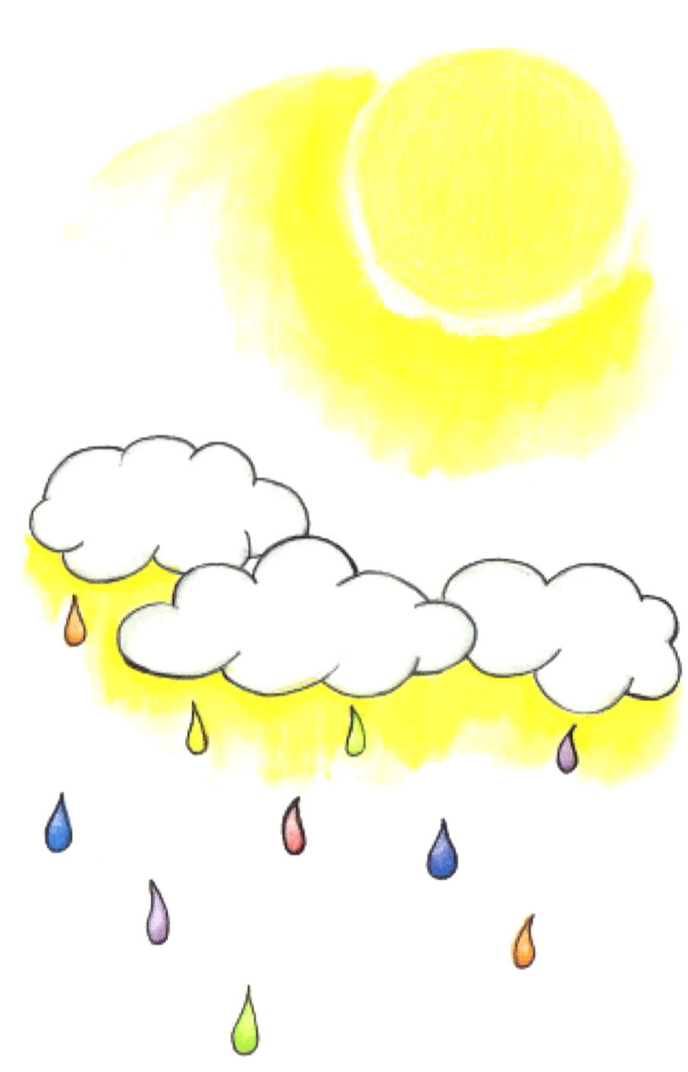

There's something else that's just not right.

Raindrops with colors, oh what a bright sight.

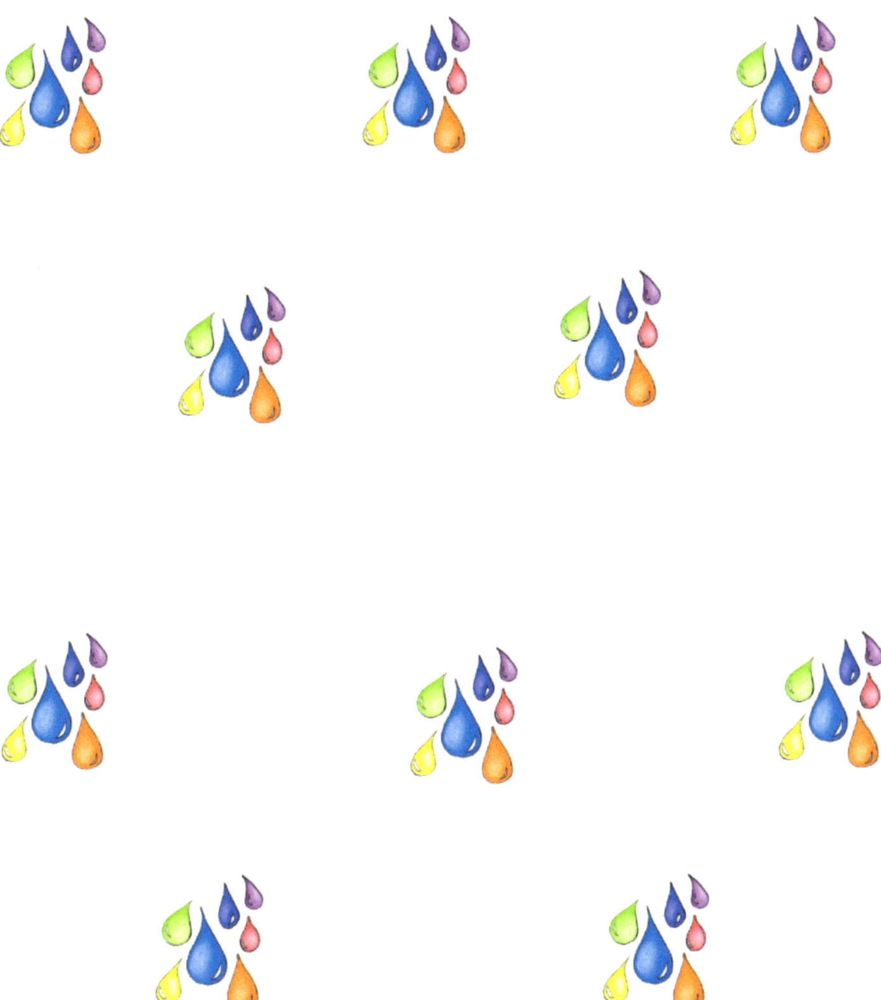

Let's meet some new friends right now.
They'll help us figure this out somehow.

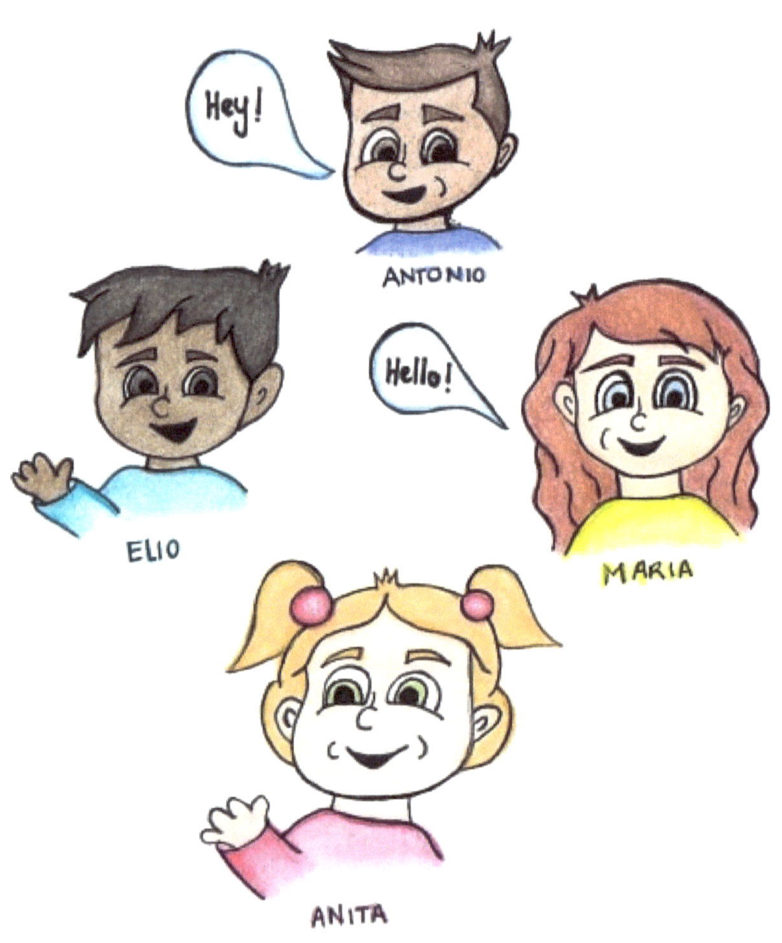

Antonio plays soccer with Elio his brother.
The ball flies fast, kicked one to another.

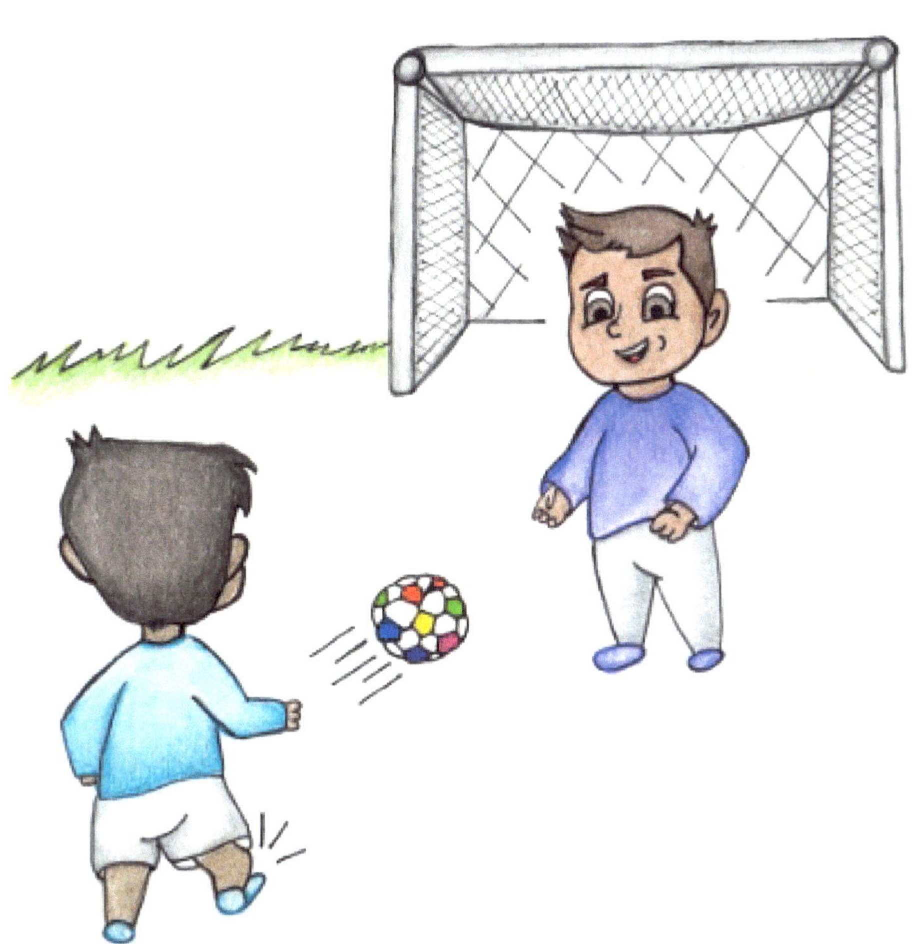

Anita and Maria, so speedy they run.
Anita scores a goal. Yeah, they won!!

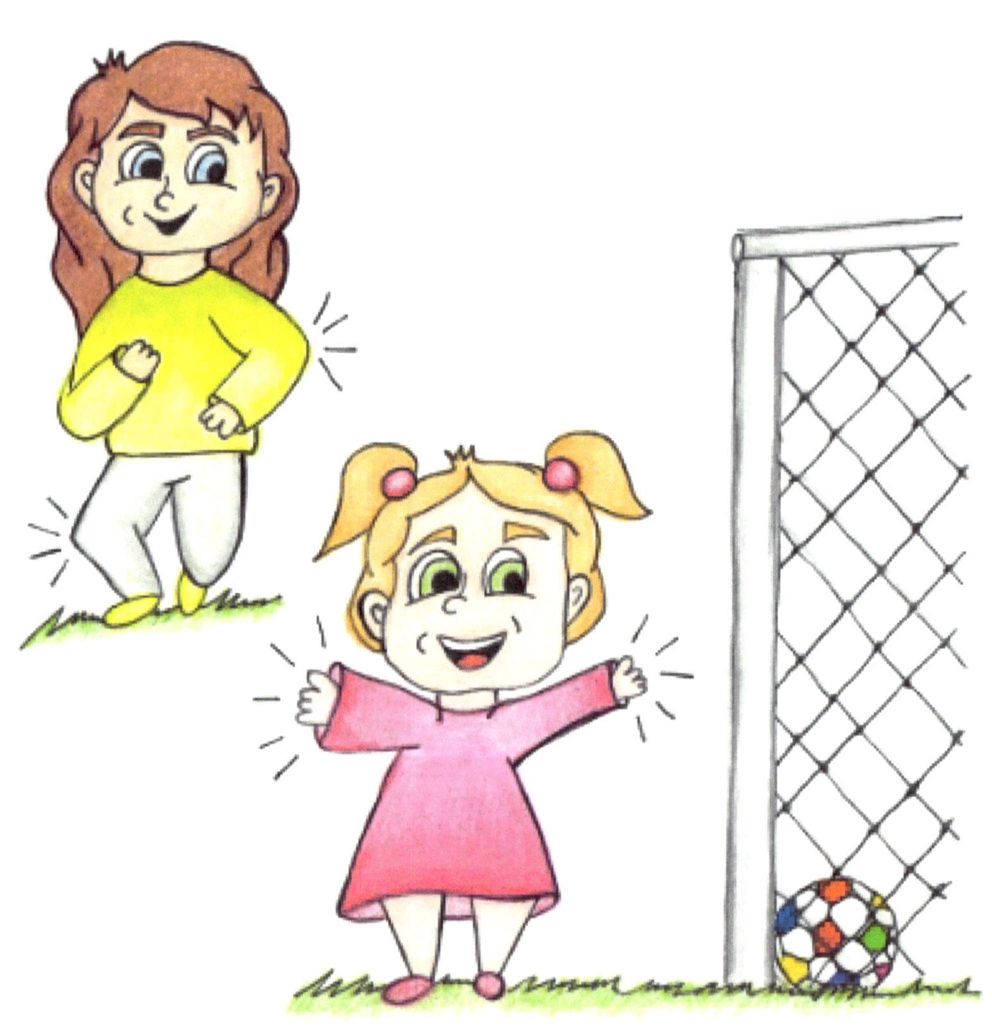

The four friends love to play TOGETHER.

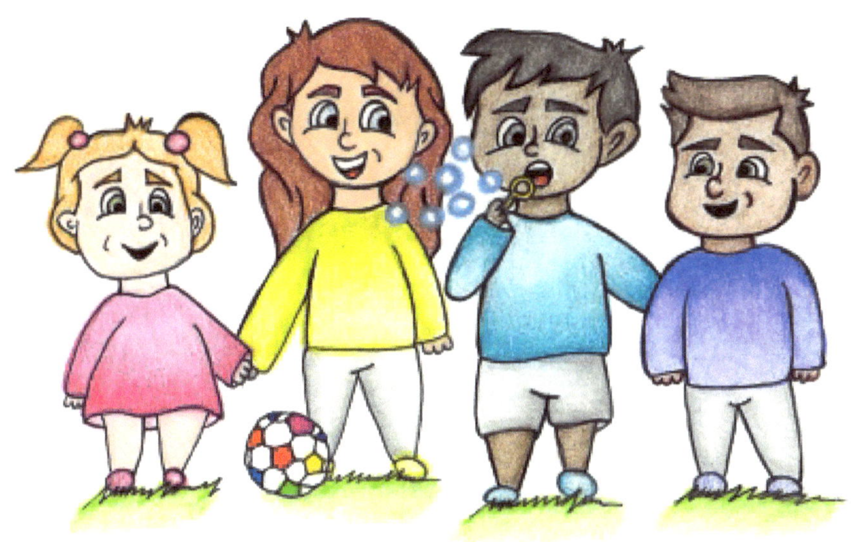

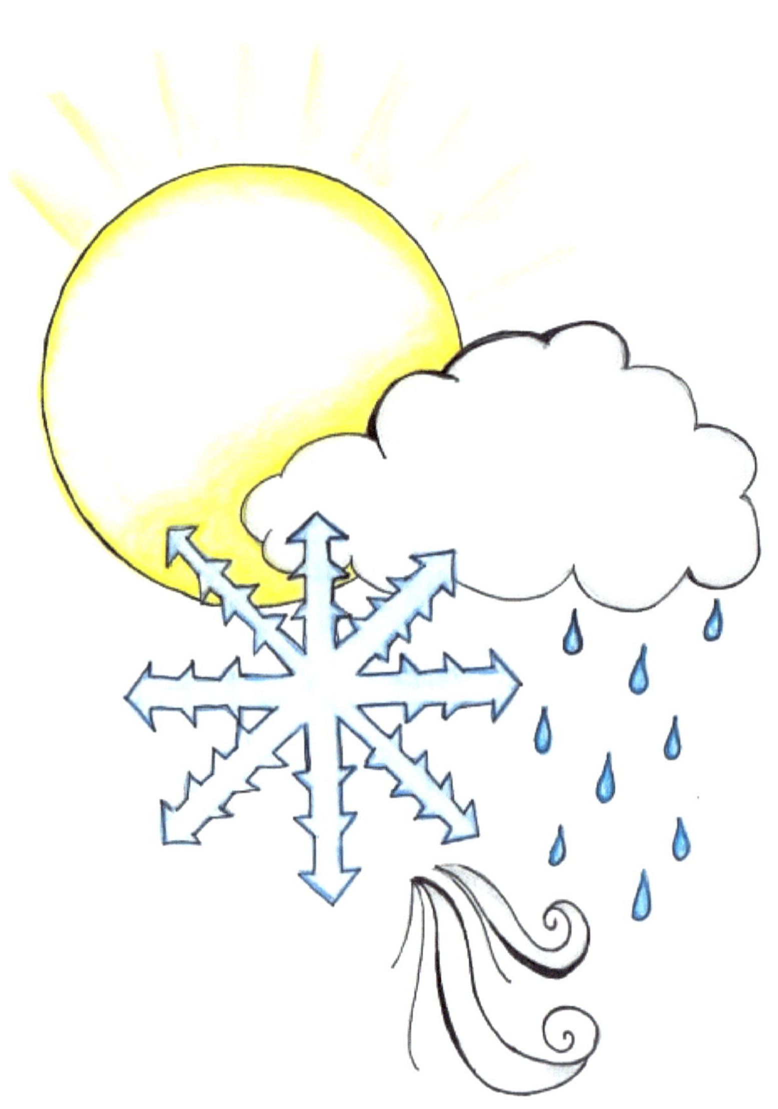

On blue sky days, they go for a ride.

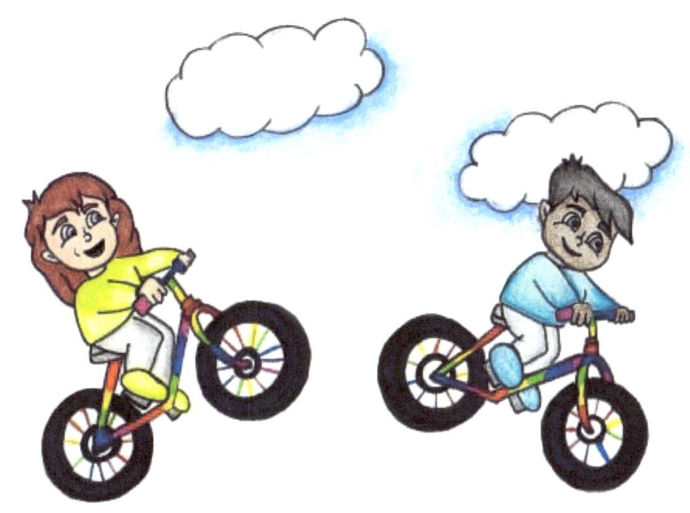

When raindrops fall, build a fort inside.

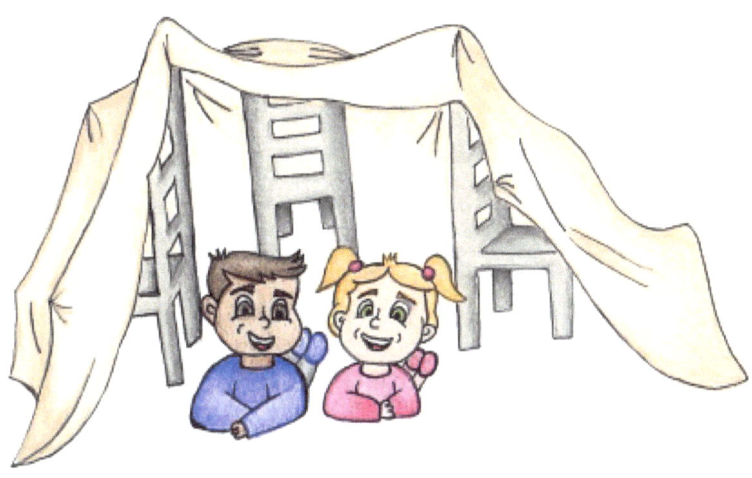

Snowballs are fun when they're home from school.

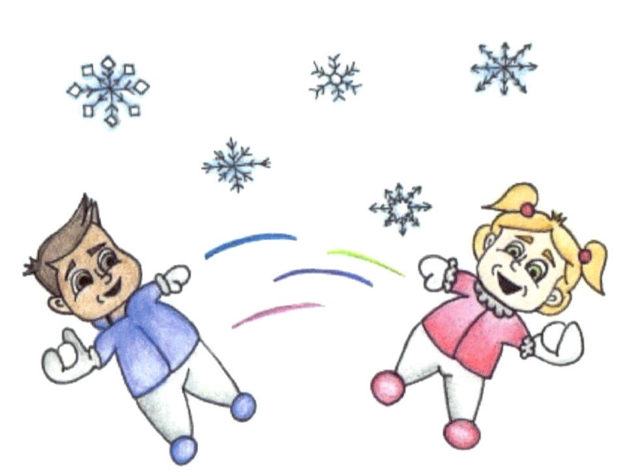

On summer days, splash at the beach or pool.

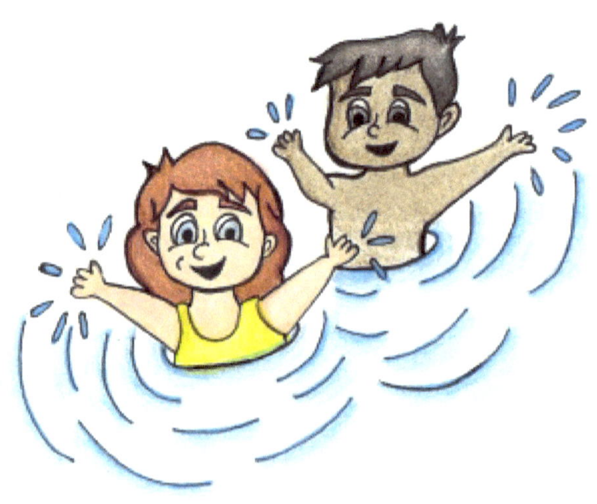

The boys are excited to run and play.

Ready and dressed to enjoy the day.

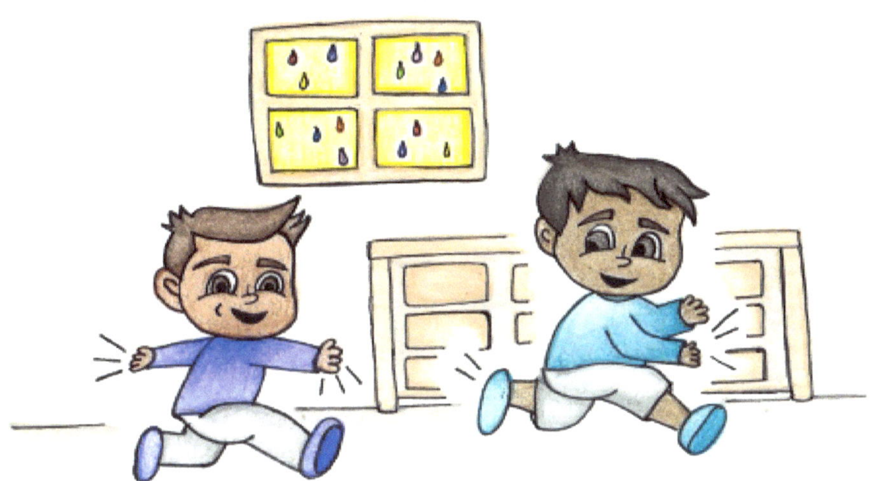

Before they go, just one more task.

"Don't forget to wear your mask!"

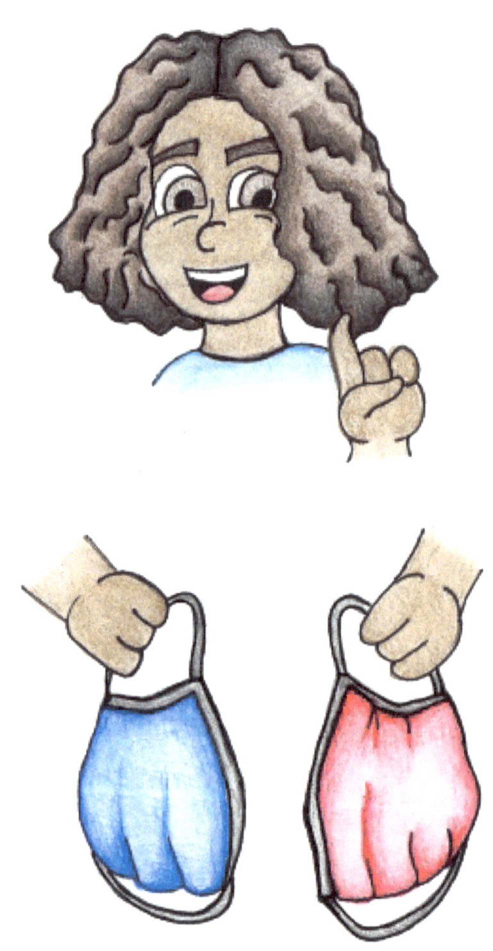

Antonio wondered and so he asked,
"Why do we need to wear a mask?
We've never had to wear this before.
Not with friends, to school or the store"

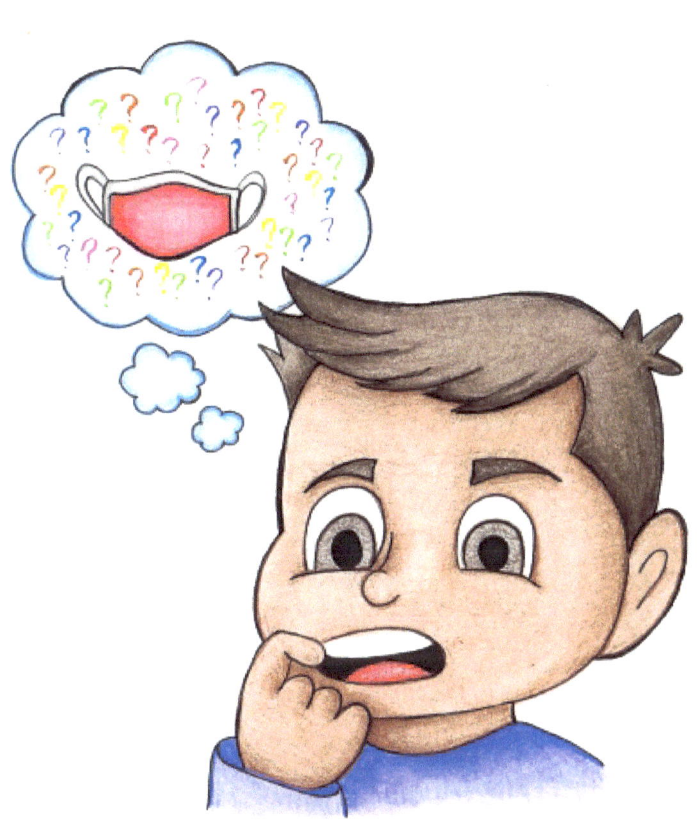

"There's a virus spreading in the world right now.
We need to stay healthy and this is how."
"Masks block germs from your mouth and nose.
Luckily these germs don't get into your toes."

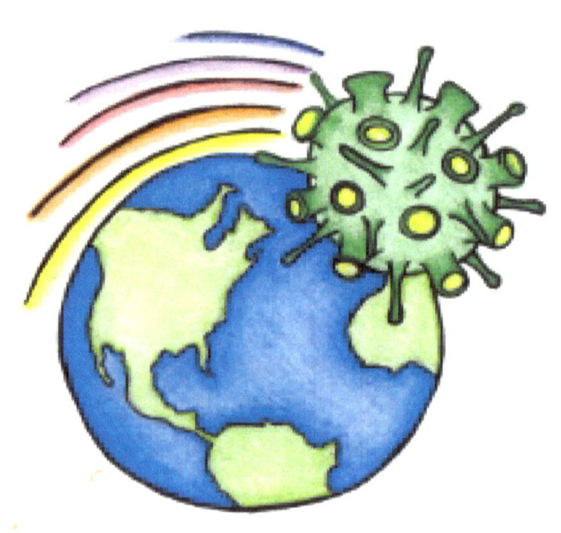

Before the boys' mom could say anymore,

The wind blew Magical Morgan in the door.

Morgan said "Abracadabra" and before they knew,
The boys had on masks, Antonio's red and Elio's blue.

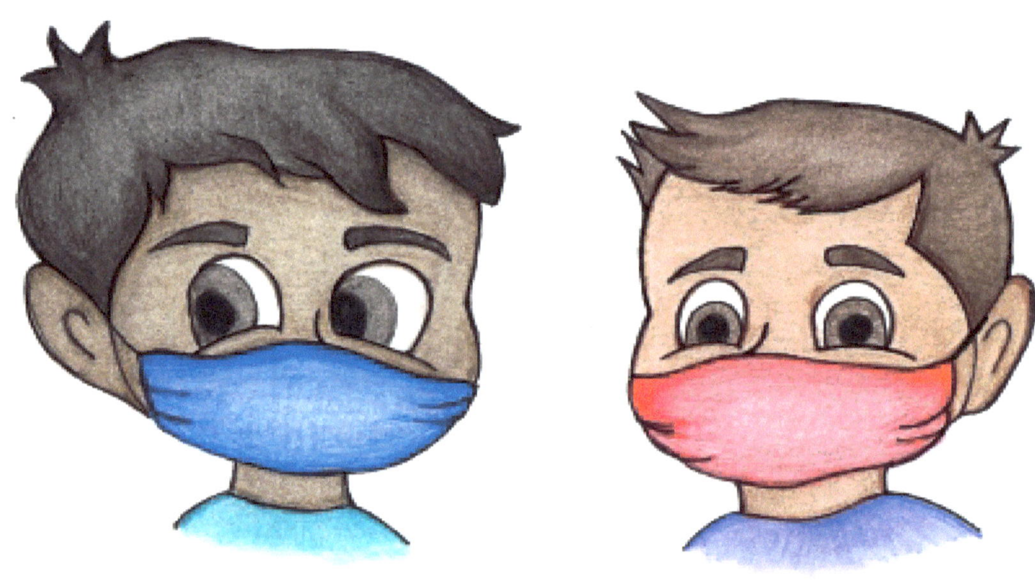

Morgan started to move with jiggles and wiggles.

"Enjoy a day with me, we'll have some giggles."

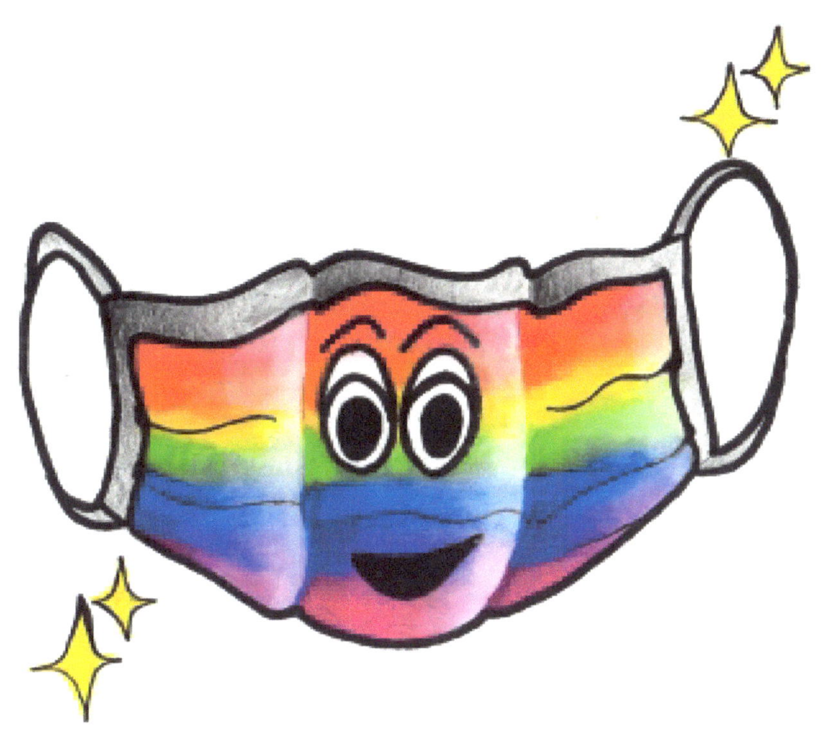

"You'll need to believe in magic just as I do."
With an "Abracadabra" out the door they flew.

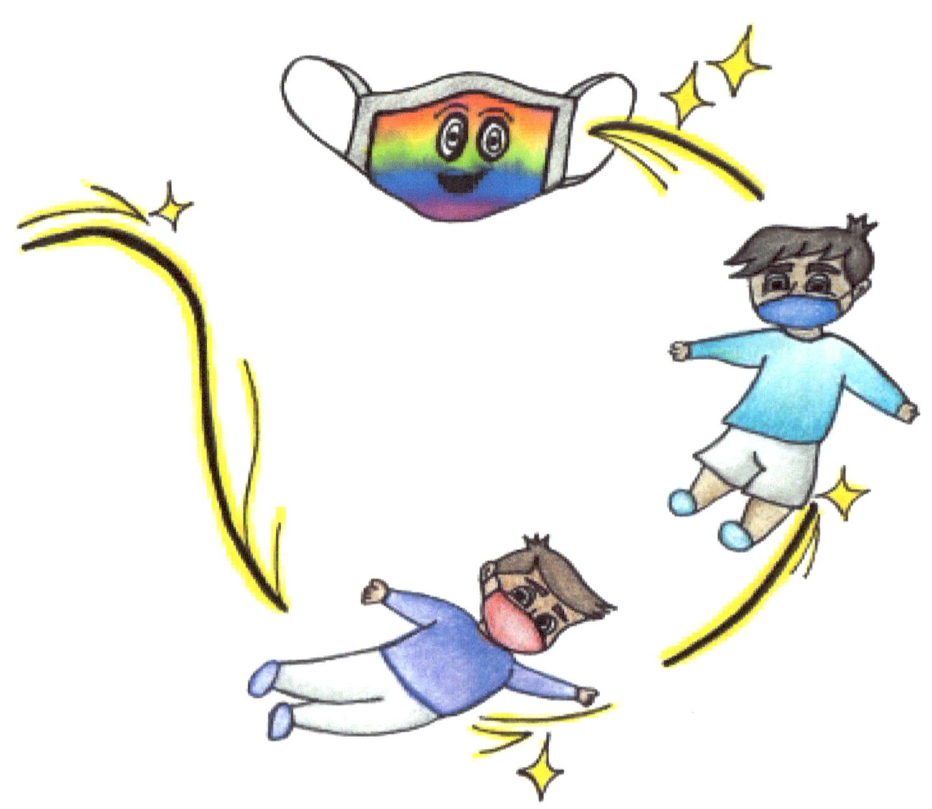

Anita and Maria had climbed an apple tree.
Now they're in a jam not sure what's to be.
Luckily for them Magical Morgan was in the air.
In the blink of an eye the mask could fly there.

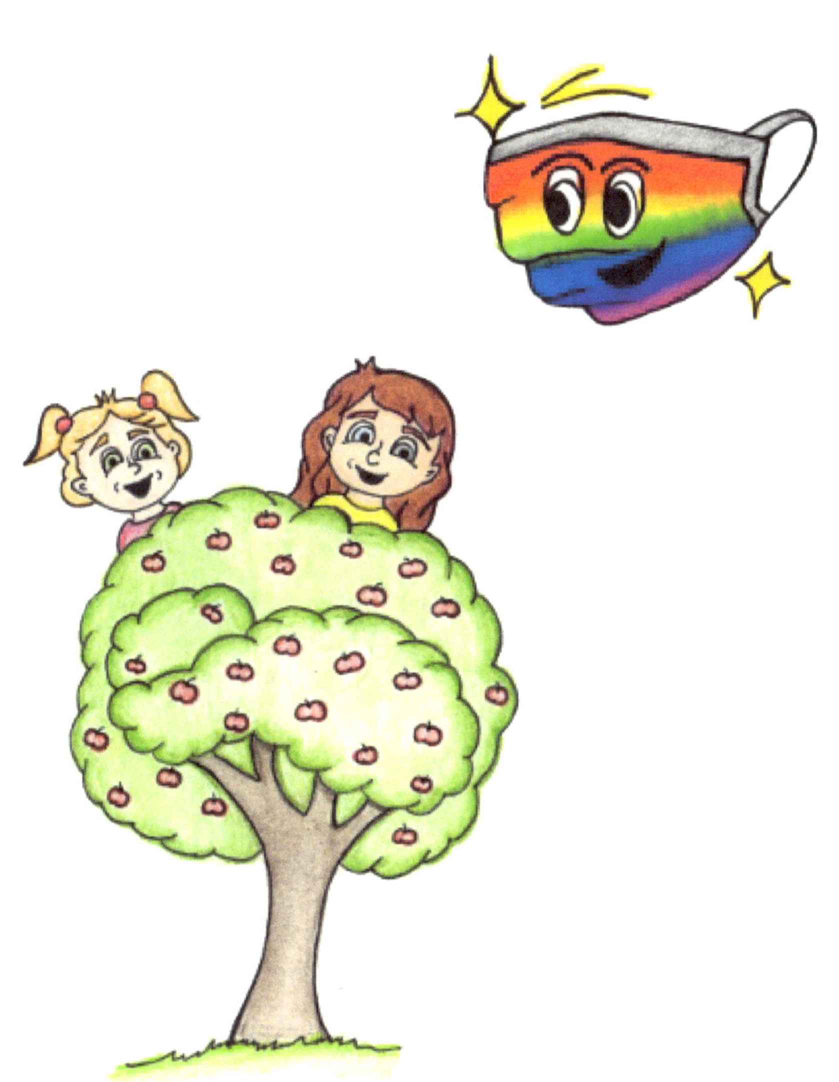

Magical Morgan jiggled and wiggled. The girls had a ride.

They happily held their heads high with pride.

Anita and Maria love adventures and to reach for a star.

Riding Magical Morgan was fun, they hoped to go far.

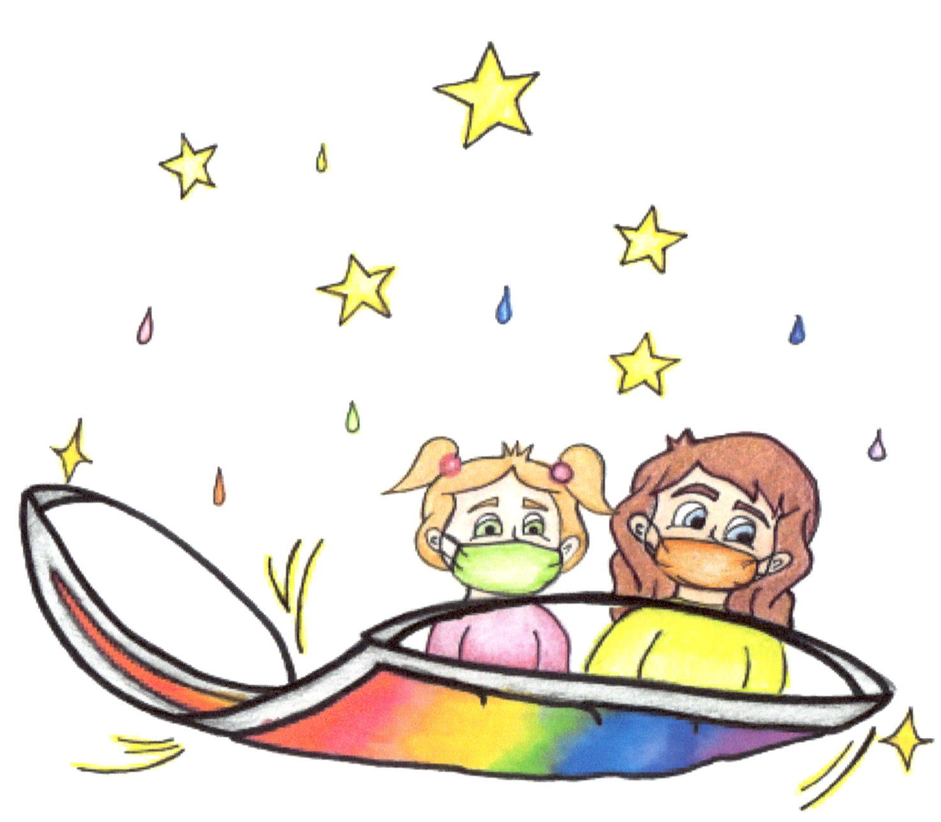

Antonio, Elio, Anita and Maria were finally TOGETHER.
Antonio said, "Look! Are the raindrops changing to feathers?"
Maria said, "No, not feathers. They're masks flying around!"
The friends jumped and laughed and rolled on the ground.

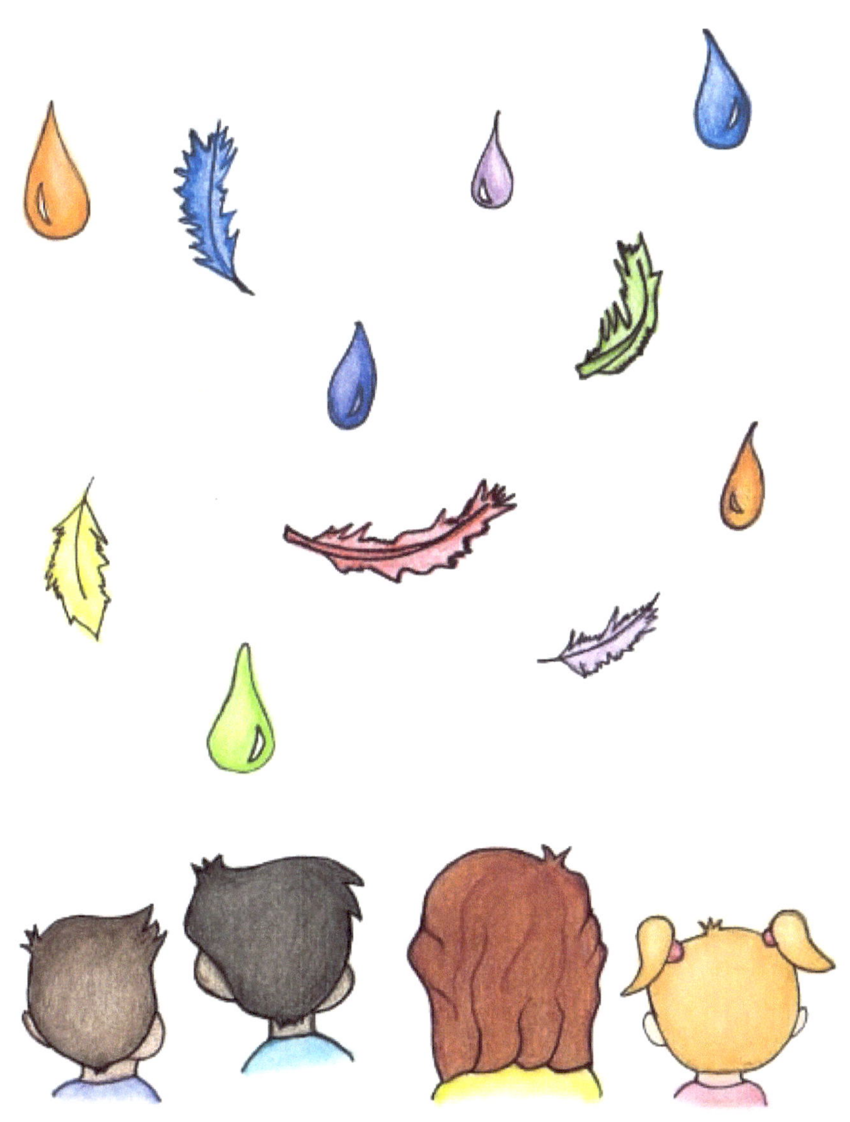

Anita gave each of her friends something to do.
"Let's sort all the colors, the red from the blue.
The orange, yellow, purple, each had its place.
Elio sorted fastest. He always likes to race.

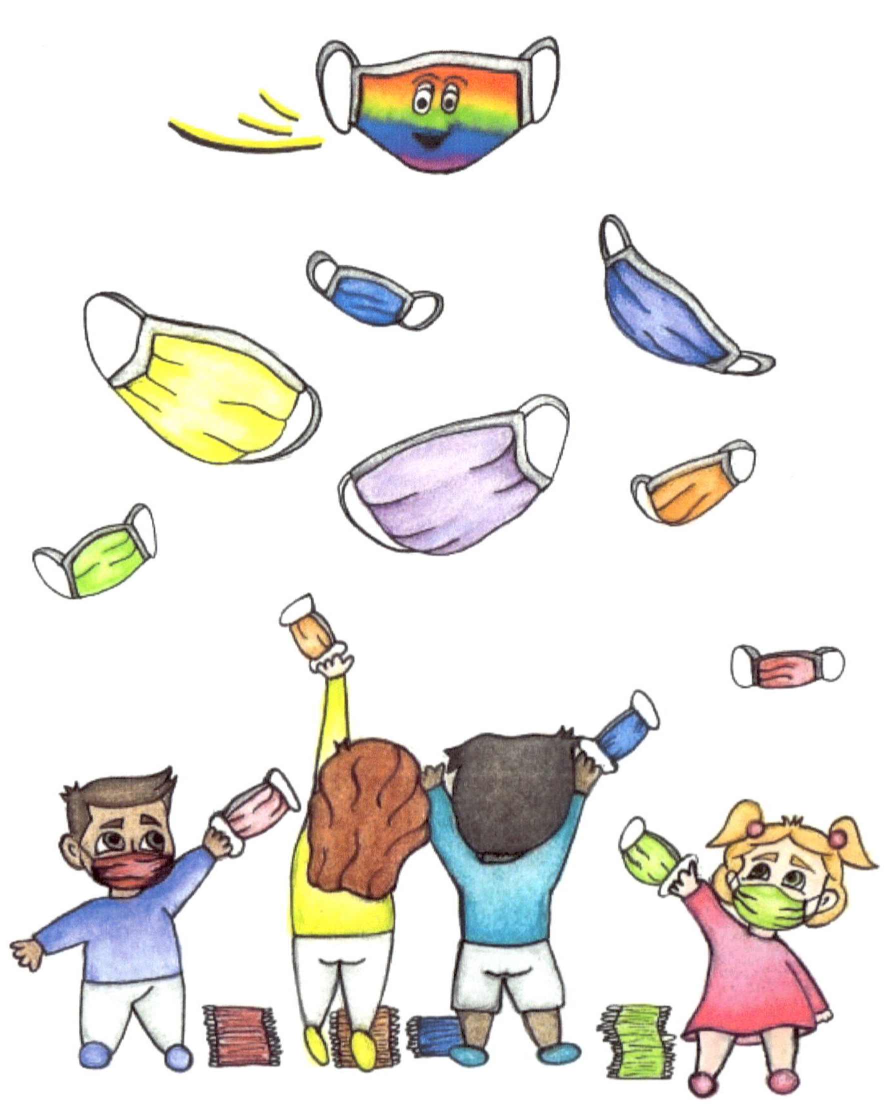

With an "Abracadabra," a rainbow crossed the sky.

An arc of colorful masks shone bright and high.

They now knew why the rain had so many colors--

To grow into masks for all sisters and brothers.

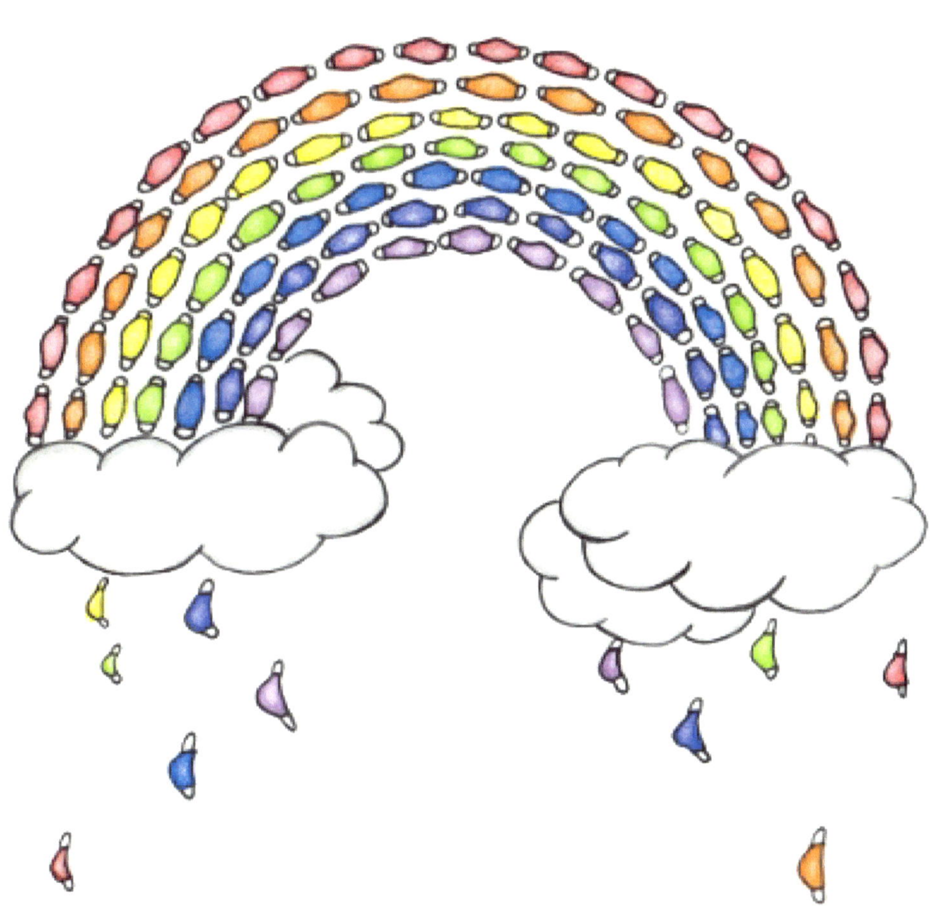

People came out to see this brilliant sight,
Which filled their hearts with great delight.

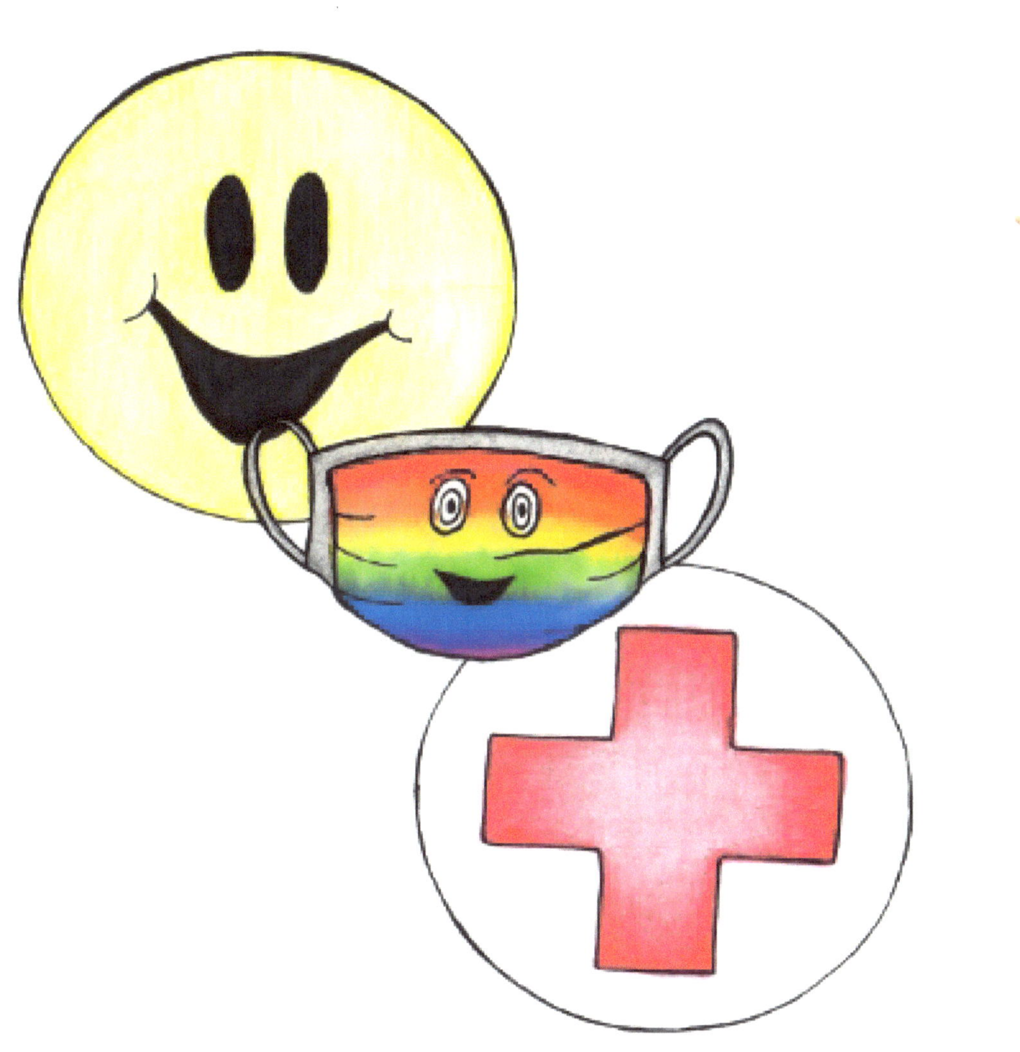

Magical Morgan said. "There's a mask for all to wear.

Be healthy and happy and always take care."

Everything Magical Morgan did was very clever.

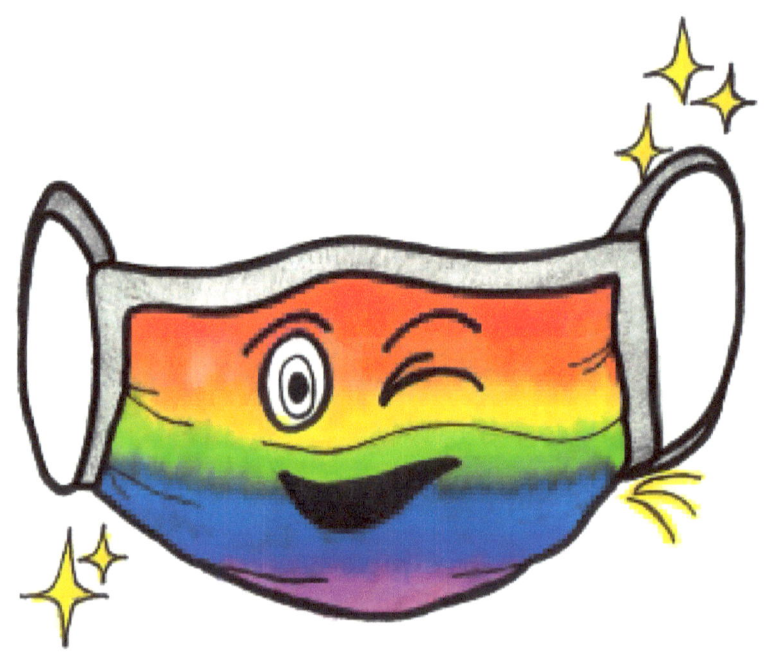

Big and small held hands to be friends forever,
TOGETHER.

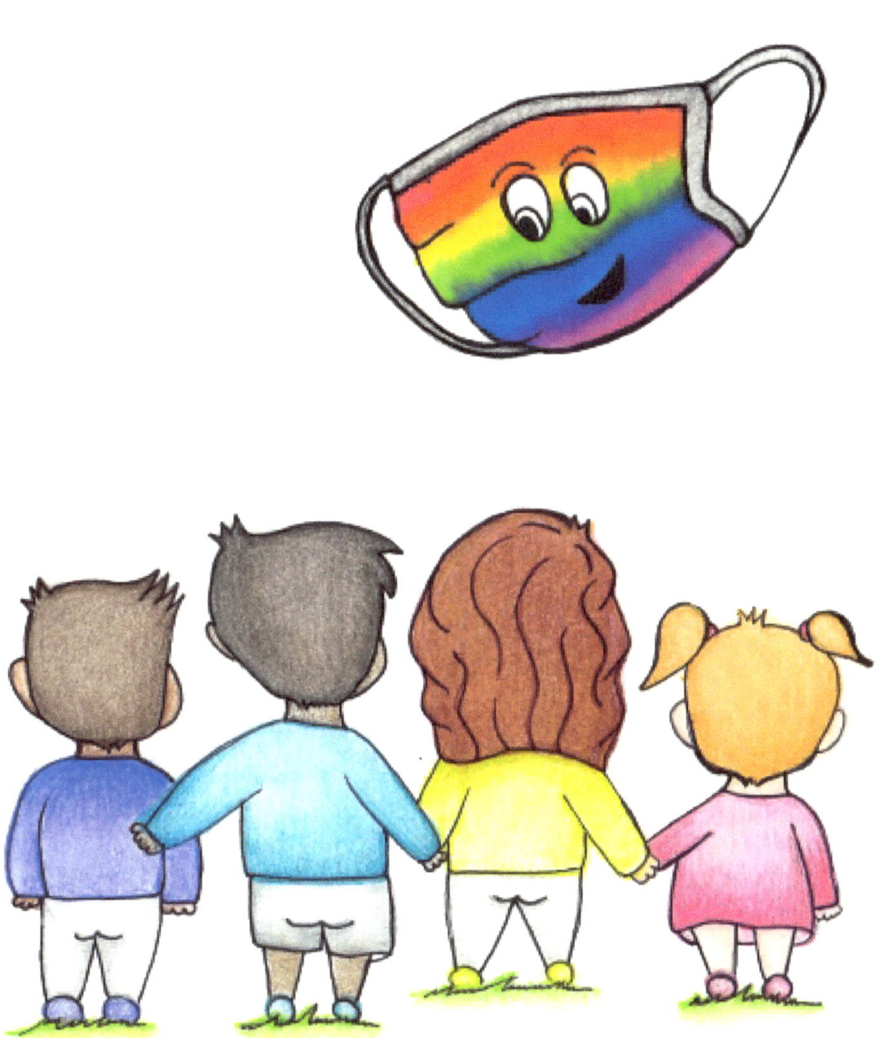